How To Be A Thin Person:
The 35 Essential Habits of Thin People

Robert Roi

ISBN-13: 978-1499326611

ISBN-10: 1499326610

℥ CONTENTS ℥

🏃 Introduction 🏃

It is obvious enough if you think about it – only fat people go on diets!

Your gut response to this statement of the blindingly obvious may well be that this is because thin people don't need to go on diets. However, I want to suggest that something more profound is going on. I want to suggest that we have the relationship between overweight people and diets the wrong way round. It is not that fat people need to go on diets; it is that diets are partly why millions of people are overweight.

The evidence for this is straightforward enough. The overwhelming majority of people who go on diets end up heavier afterward than they were at the start. The process goes something like this (and this is true for just about every fad or celebrity diet you have ever heard of):

○ The diet will recommend a change of diet and/or less calorie intake – this usually involves substituting highly calorific foods (especially sugar) with healthy alternatives (usually fresh fruit and veg)l; some kind of supplement shake; or nothing at all (i.e., fasting)

- The shift in food intake results in a dramatic weight loss during the first month
- After 4-6 weeks the rate of weight loss slows and eventually levels out
- Within 6 months the weight starts to go on once more (often because dieters lapse back to old eating habits)
- Six to 12 months after going on the diet, weight gain has overtaken the weight at the beginning of the diet.

This "yo-yo" dieting process is now so well documented in the scientific literature as well as the popular media that we might reasonably argue that any doctor who tells a patient to go on a diet should be struck-off for malpractice!

Of course, not everyone who goes on a diet experiences this yo-yo effect. Around five percent of dieters manage to keep the weight off; and that is great... *for them.* The problem is that we have tended to focus on them when looking at what the rest of us can do to lose weight.

We've all seen those "before and after" advertisements where someone has managed to shed several stones, and now looks fantastic[1]. The

---

[1] What we don't get to see is whether these lucky few manage to keep the weight off for the rest of their lives or whether they slip back into their old fat habits after the photographs have been taken. And, of course,

implication is always that *you too* could achieve the same results. This is a myth that causes misery and low self-esteem, because the diets that succeed in five percent of people also fail 95 percent of the time. What this means in practice is that if you or I follow the same approach, the odds are 19 to 1 for us ending up heavier!

By looking at the minority of fat people who manage to get thin, we are actually setting ourselves up to fail. However, there is another group of people who succeed in maintaining a healthy weight week-in, week-out... *Thin people*!

I should qualify this. Among thin people there are two groups:

1. Thin-fat people
2. Thin-thin people

Thin-fat people appear to be healthy because their weight is within healthy parameters. However, they may be thin on the outside, but they are fat on the inside – their internal organs are surrounded by the dangerous visceral fat that leads to illness. In many ways, this group are at greater risk of developing metabolic syndrome illnesses because –

---

many of the photographs are doctored using programmes like Photoshop. Indeed, some of the most unscrupulous advertisers have even swapped the before and after images around!

unlike overweight people – they don't know they have a problem[2].

Thin-thin people are healthy both on the inside and the outside because they have a healthy approach to physical activity and diet. But more importantly, they exercise a high degree of willpower.

If you wish to lose weight and stay lighter and healthier, don't go on a diet – instead, learn to follow the example of these thin-thin people. In this book, I will show you how. In the first part, I have set out the how thin-thin people approach physical activity. In the second part I examine their relationship with food. Finally, I explain how they maintain strong willpower; something we can all learn with practice.

---

[2] At the time of writing, it is only possible to measure visceral fat using very expensive fMRI scans. However, some new abdominal fat scanners are coming onto the market in the next year, which will allow clinics to offer you a reasonably accurate measurement of internal fat.

🎿 One: Thin people are active people 🎿

Human beings have evolved in the last 100,000 years.   For sure, we have a good deal of technology and we have harnessed fossil fuels to provide abundant energy.   However, we are no more intelligent and no different physically to our hunter-gathering ancestors.

Why am I telling you this?   Because it has huge ramifications for modern humans' approaches to physical activity.

If you suggested working out, going for a run, or going to the gym to one of your hunter-gathering ancestors, she would look at you as if you had completely lost the plot.   Physical activity is what she did in the course of her everyday life just to survive.   Her problem was not finding the time to get physical, it was finding the energy (calories) to allow her to function.   In those mid-winter days when sufficient calories were not available, her body would begin to shut down in order to preserve the few calories that she had managed to store in the form of body fat.

So we have evolved not to *burn* extra calories but to *store* them. This has two consequences in the modern world, where our problem is an over-abundance of calories. First, we have to fight against our bodies' natural default in order to be more active. Second, we have to guard against our bodies' inclination to take on extra calories and to take more rest after we have been active.

In this sense, overweight people are "normal". It is thin-thin people who are extraordinary in their ability to manage their biology. And it is important to realise that – whether by accident or design – they are managing. Often, they have used their ability to think, learn, and to change behaviour – abilities we all have – to overcome their natural inclinations. This means that you too can learn to manage your biology by adopting new habits.

So how do thin-thin people differ from overweight people in their physical habits?

🏃 Habit one: thin people fidget

When you were a child you were probably told off for fidgeting. Children were supposed to be "seen but not heard", and good girls and boys learned to sit patiently. Indeed, in the modern world, children that fidget too much risk being diagnosed with some over-medicalised condition like ADHD. But children are meant to fidget – it is part of the way they develop the muscle and bone strength that they will require as adults.

While most of us had our fidgeting habit disciplined out of us as youngsters, thin-thin people are always moving – often annoyingly so. Their feet are tapping, their heads are nodding, and they move their hands and arms when they speak. Research suggests that someone who fidgets will burn the same number of calories as someone who takes a brisk one-mile walk every day.

While much of this fidgeting is ingrained habit, it is possible to copy. You could get up from your desk or armchair and walk around once every 30 minutes or every hour. You could learn to do more things standing up. Try walking around while you are talking on the phone. Don't just listen to music; tap your feet, swing your arms or dance.

Habit two: thin people take the stairs

Most of us have learned to choose the sedentary option when presented with a choice. We drive to the shops when we could walk. We sit when we could stand. We park as close as we can get to the shopping centre entrance. We take the elevator and the escalator. We keep the phone to hand so we don't have to get up to answer it. We eat out or eat ready-meals rather than cook from scratch.

No doubt you can add some of your own calorie-conserving habits to the list.

Thin-thin people simply do not choose in this way. They take the stairs, walk rather than drive, and park at the far end of the car park. In short, while the majority of us default to conserving calories, they always choose to burn them. And, once again, the cumulative effect of these choices is that they burn the equivalent of another brisk one-mile walk.

🏃 Habit three: thin people walk after meals

The chances are that when you have eaten, you feel full and lethargic. You just want to sit still for 15-30 minutes "while your food goes down". This is exactly what your body evolved to do when it couldn't be sure of its next meal. By resting after meals, your body could avoid burning calories and store them for later as fat instead.

Thin-thin people do the opposite. They have got into the habit of gentle exercise – usually walking and moving around – immediately after eating. This causes their bodies to burn the calories that are stored in the muscles as glucose. This, in turn, results in the calories they have just consumed being sent to the muscles rather than being laid down as fat.

⚡ Habit four: thin people know how to rev up their metabolism

There is a myth that thin people have higher metabolism than fat people. In fact, the opposite is true. Fat people's bodies have to work harder than thin people's, so their heart rate, blood pressure and the rate at which they burn calories are all faster. The problem is that fat people are inclined to feel hungry as a result, and are likely to eat far too many calories.

Thin-thin people will often use foods (see habit 16) and caffeine to speed up their metabolism. They may also engage in short-duration/high-intensity physical activities like circuit training or 30 second sprints within a regular 20 minute walking, jogging, swimming or cycling activity.

While you are losing weight, it is better to engage in simple physical activities like walking, cycling, jogging and swimming. However, short-duration/high-intensity physical activties may be an option to help you maintain a healthy weight once you have achieved it[3].

---

[3] It should go without saying that if you are very obese and/or you have any physical health conditions, you should see your doctor and get advice on the type and duration of physical activity that you engage in.

🏃 Habit five: thin people exercise with someone (a little) fitter than them

Having an exercise buddy can make the difference between actually *doing* exercise and just sitting round thinking about doing it. Once you have made an arrangement to meet up with your buddy, you are much more likely to do it than make excuses.

Thin-thin people add to this by selecting an exercise buddy who is a little[4] bit fitter than they are. This is because the aim of exercise is to increase fitness and stamina. When you are playing catch-up with your exercise buddy, you will always put that extra bit of effort in.

🏃 Habit six: thin people rest up

When we get tired and/or stressed, our bodies can mistake the low energy sensation for hunger. This is especially so if we are in a situation where we have to keep going. This usually means that we take on additional calories when we should be resting.

---

[4] If you choose someone who is much fitter than you are, they will leave you so far behind that there is a strong risk that you will give up. If you work with someone less fit than you, the danger is that you will put less effort in than you need to.

Thin-thin people tend to be more in tune with the difference between genuine hunger and the low-energy sensations associated with tiredness and stress. As such, rather than eating, they are much more likely to take five minutes out to rest and relax.

🏃 Habit Seven: thin people sleep well

In the same way as general tiredness and stress, poor and insufficient sleep creates a low-energy sensation that is mistaken for hunger. The tendency to eat more when you are tired is not just to do with your body's desire to take on additional calories; it is also to do with the effect of low energy on the parts of the brain that give you willpower (see habits 17 to 35).

Thin-thin people tend to enjoy more and better quality sleep. In part, this is because being overweight impairs sleep. However, it is also because they have developed a series of good habits that are collectively known as "sleep hygiene". These include not consuming caffeine in the evening; avoiding screens (TV, computers, phones, etc) in the hour before bed; keeping the bedroom clean, cool (not cold), dark and fragrant; and banishing clocks from the bedroom[5].

---

[5] We have produced a Life Surfing guide on *Getting to Sleep* which explores these issues in more depth.

⚡Two: Thin people eat healthily ⚡

It goes without saying that thin-thin people eat healthily. But what, exactly, does this mean?

As with physical activity, being healthy means fighting against your nature. Our ancestors had to survive in a harsh environment where energy was in short-supply. As such, we evolved a taste (bordering on an addiction) for high-density sources of calories. In nature, these come from two sources – fats and sugars. Whenever our ancestors encountered fat or sugar, they were pre-programmed to gorge on them. The aim was to store as much energy as possible (in the form of fat), so that this would be available at a later time when food was scarce.

In our contemporary food-rich environment, this natural inclination to gorge on high-fat and high-sugar foods is proving catastrophic for millions of people. So much so that we have had to develop an expensive public health education system to advise us on what we should and should not eat… and in what quantities.

In fact, several of the healthy eating rules promoted by government and much of the medical profession turn out to be wrong outside the laboratory. Two of these messages are very important for those who want to get thin... and stay thin:

o "Low fat is healthy", and
o "All calories are equal".

The government and the medical profession tell us that our diets should be "low-fat/high-fibre". No surprise, then, that the supermarkets are full of "healthy" low fat foods. The trouble is that low-fat is unhealthy because genuinely low-fat or fat-free foods taste dry and bland. Anyone unfortunate enough to have tried the first veggie burgers (which tasted – and looked – like cork floor tiles) knows what this is like! It is the fat in cheese, chocolate and cakes that makes them so appealing.

Removing fat from foods was relatively simple for the food industry. Creating low-fat foods that people wanted to buy was much more challenging. In the end, the only thing they could do to make low-fat and fat-free foods tasty was to make them sweet. And that meant adding sugar – usually in the form of High Fructose Corn Syrup (which is cheaper and three times as sweet as white sugar).

So while there is a basic truth in the government/medical message – that we shouldn't load up on fats – we have more often ended up dangerously overloading our systems with sugar. And we now know that sugar (actually the fructose within sugar) is many times more dangerous than fat.

This brings us to the second common misconception about food: that all calories are equal. According to both the government and the food industry, we should consume a set number of calories every day – on average 2,500 for men and 2,000 for women. It doesn't matter where these calories come from so long as we burn as many calories as we consume.

The simplistic government message is based on the physics of closed systems in which energy cannot disappear, it can only change form. If you eat 400 calories then you must either burn them or store them – you cannot simply make them disappear. But common sense tells us that this message is plain wrong. Consuming 400 calories in a large glass of cola is going to affect us in a very different way to consuming 400 calories from a (large) plate of carrots!

The human body is not a simple closed system, and it has more than two choices (burn or store) when dealing with calories. A litre bottle of cola contains roughly 400 calories in the form of sugars (mainly High Fructose Corn Syrup). That's equivalent to about 28 teaspoons of sugar. When this hits your stomach, it is quickly broken down into two chemicals – glucose, which produces a blood sugar spike that interferes with your insulin levels and disrupts the hormone *Leptin* which tells your brain you have enough energy – and fructose, an alien substance that can only be metabolised by the liver, which converts it to fat. Because your stomach doesn't recognise cola as food, you continue to feel hungry afterwards. It will do nothing to curb your appetite, so the 400 calories will most likely be additional to your normal daily intake.

Now consider the (large[6]) plate of carrots. They contain the same number of calories, but your body will deal with them in a very different way. First, they are a greater volume than your stomach, so you will feel full long before you finish eating them (you will have to consume them in several sittings). Also, they are high in fibre, so your body will have to work to get the energy (calories) from them. Indeed, as with most fibrous foods, your body will not be able to process all of the calories; some will simply pass through your body.

Your digestive system will break down the carrots, but much more slowly than the couple of seconds

---

[6] Depending on their size, 400 calories will be around 35 carrots!

that it took to separate the glucose and fructose in the glass of cola. As a result, there will not be a sugar spike to interfere with your insulin levels or to block the leptin signal that tells your brain you've got enough energy. Your body will break the carrots down into glucose, some of which will be used to provide your cells with energy immediately and some will be stored in the muscles. Crucially, carrots neither contain nor break down into fructose, so you will only store energy (glucose) as fat if you have more than enough calories already.

If your gut instinct was that not all calories are equal, you were dead right!

The broader public health advice to eat a diet that is high in fibre and low in fat, salt and sugar is more useful. In practice it means that most of the food we eat should be in the form of vegetables and fruits. Our carbohydrates should be complex (whole grains) rather than refined (e.g., sugar, white bread, pasta, rice and flour). Meat and fat should only ever be a small addition to a meal, never a meal in itself.

Whether by accident or design, thin-thin people know and act upon this.

𝓔 Habit eight: thin people eat breakfast

Breakfast (i.e., breaking the fast) is the most important meal of the day. However, in our busy 24-hour society, there is a huge temptation to snooze in bed until the very last minute before heading off on the daily commute. If we eat at all, it is likely to be a quick, sugary snack washed down with coffee while we are on the move.

The result is that we experience a quick and unhealthy blood sugar spike followed rapidly by feeling hungry again. This usually means snacking (on sugary foods) to keep us going until lunchtime.

Thin-thin people always make time for a sit down breakfast, even if this means getting to bed an hour earlier at night. And breakfast for thin-thin people will be slow-release foods such as oats or scrambled eggs on toast that will maintain their energy levels throughout the morning.

𝓔 Habit nine: thin people don't skip meals

It is tempting to imagine that skipping a meal will help you reduce the number of calories you consume. And it is easy to skip a meal if you lead a busy lifestyle.

However, the evidence is against you.

While your conscious mind knows that you are going to have a meal later on, your body doesn't know this. As far as your body is concerned, you are facing starvation and it needs to conserve energy. So you are likely to get tired and irritable. You are also likely to develop cravings for high-energy foods, and will probably end up over-eating at your next meal.

Thin-thin people stick to a regular series of mealtimes in order to regulate properly the way their bodies consume and process food.

🏃 Habit ten: thin people drink water

There is a growing body of evidence that overweight people mistake the sensation of thirst for the sensation of hunger. The result is that when we need a drink, we end up eating instead.

Thin-thin people are much more likely to avoid dehydration by drinking the recommended six glasses (about 2 litres) of water (or other non-alcoholic beverages – but not soda) per day.

🏃 Habit eleven: thin people eat protein with at least two of their meals

Protein is essential for building and repairing muscle. It also suppresses feelings of hunger.

Unfortunately, too many of us consume protein in the form of fatty meats, cheeses and processed ready meals that are also high in calories.

Thin-thin people by contrast prepare and eat meals containing a portion (about the size of a computer mouse) of lean meat, fish or eggs. This helps them avoid the temptation to seek an unhealthy energy boost (like a bar of chocolate) between meals.

⚡ Habit twelve: thin people favour bulky foods

Recent research suggests that the "calorie density" of foods is important to whether they aid or prevent weight loss. Low density foods have a large ratio of water and fibre per calorie. These include most vegetables and fruit, water-based soups and stews, and cooked whole grains.

Thin-thin people often begin a meal with a filling soup or a salad, which causes mind and body to feel fuller. As a result, they eat less and do not feel a need for dessert.

⚡ Habit thirteen: thin people switch white carbs to brown

Calorie density is particularly important when choosing carbohydrates. Brown – wholemeal – sources of carbohydrates (like rice, pasta and bread) are higher in fibre than white – refined – versions. Also, at the cheaper end of the market, many white carbohydrates contain added sugar which makes them even more calorie dense.

Thin-thin people will choose brown/wholemeal carbohydrates because these are also more filling than white carbs.

🏃 Habit fourteen: thin people eat healthy snacks

Because of their other eating habits, thin-thin people are much less likely to feel the need for a snack between meals. However, where the rest of us might be tempted by a high-calorie snack like a bar of chocolate or a muesli bar with added sugar, thin-thin people are much more likely to graze on vegetables like celery or carrots, high-fibre fruits like apples or bananas, or turn to a small portion of seeds and nuts.

🏃 Habit fifteen: thin people chew thoroughly

A combination of the pace of life and the vast array of distractions (TV, computers, phones, etc) have speeded the pace at which most of us eat. Many workers "desk dine" – i.e., we are encouraged to eat at our work stations; often while continuing to interact with our computer screens. This means that far too many of us end up gulping down our food without chewing it properly.

This is a public health catastrophe. It can take 15 to 20 minutes for the hormones produced by a full stomach to signal to the brain that you have eaten enough. Not chewing properly means that you have gulped down more than enough food before your system has caught up. One result is that far too many of us will be tempted to eat dessert, or wash our food down with a soda.

Thin-thin people chew their food thoroughly. Many will chew each mouthful of food 20 to 30 times, savouring the flavours and textures of their food (see the section on willpower) before swallowing. In addition to the enhanced enjoyment of food that this brings, it means that thin-thin people are much more likely to feel full at the end of a meal.

Habit sixteen: thin people eat spicy foods

There is some evidence that spicy foods containing chilli peppers and garlic work to increase metabolism – causing you to burn more calories without doing extra work. Chilli peppers are particularly good because they contain a chemical called capsaicin that helps speed metabolism.

Other spices that can increase metabolism include ginger and cinnamon.

Other foods that thin-thin people eat that are thought to help increase metabolism include high-fibre fruits and vegetables, lentils, egg whites, lean meats, green tea and coffee.

Three: Thin People have willpower

There is an important psychological dimension to our relationship with food that is all too often overlooked by the diet industry. Indeed, it is essential to the corporations that profit from selling us diets that we never question the psychology of food.

The result for millions of us is that we get caught in a "willpower trap".

We have been led to believe that we need to exercise willpower in order to get thin and stay thin. There is a grain of truth to this. However, the big lie is that willpower is entirely down to us. So when we lapse, we tend to blame ourselves for our failure. The result of this self-blame is that our self-esteem plummets and our stress levels increase dramatically. We feel miserable and unloved.

And what do we do when we feel this way?

We eat!

Not only that, but we eat those foods that we have learned to associate with comfort: chocolate, cake, sweets, doughnuts, etc. And then we put on even more weight, so we beat ourselves up again, eat again, gain weight again, on and on and on.

We need to radically revise our understanding of willpower. In particular, we need to understand that a personal desire to do something (e.g., exercise more, eat healthier foods) or not do something (e.g., eat fattening foods, smoke, drink too much) is just one element of what constitutes willpower.

Willpower also requires:

- Knowledge and skills
- Friends and colleagues who act as allies not accomplices
- Someone to act (either formally or informally) as a coach, mentor or buddy
- A series of rewards and incentives (possibly balanced by forfeits)
- Control over the environment.

Most people who want to lose weight have the desire, but completely lack these other five key elements of willpower. Without them, we simply set ourselves up to fail.

Willpower has been compared to a muscle. Research has shown that willpower tires with use... and the food industry knows it!

Consider the layout of the supermarket you use. The odds are that the fresh food is up front. As soon as you walk in, you are faced with displays of fruit and vegetables. This helps to create what psychologists call the "halo effect". They know that most of their customers enter the store with a determination to exercise their willpower. So they give you what you are looking for right away. You load all of that healthy food into your trolley, and you feel really virtuous. But the feeling of virtue serves to switch off the part of your brain that exercises willpower. It is as if your brain wants to balance virtue with vice. So by the time you get further into the store, you are much more likely to add the crisps, cake, chocolate and sweets into your trolley too.

There are many other psychological tricks that supermarkets employ to negate the personal desire element of willpower. So long as they can keep convincing you that your lapses are entirely your fault, they will keep getting away with it.

Whether thin-thin people are consciously aware of what they are doing is not clear. Some will be, many will not. However, all exercise all six key elements of willpower in their relationship with food.

⚡ Habit seventeen: thin people manage stress

Stress is the number one enemy of willpower. Our ancestors evolved just three responses to danger – fight, flight or freeze. None of these require the ability to think rationally, so the blood supply to the front of the brain (the bit that does the thinking and exercises willpower) is switched off and blood (and the glucose – energy – it contains) is diverted to the muscles.

In the modern world, most stressful situations can only be resolved by thinking. However, if we become stressed, we are lost. Our willpower drops to zero!

It should come as no surprise that supermarkets are laid out in a way that makes us feel like rats in a maze, or that bright lights, background noise, artificial smells and trolley jams at pinch points are all designed to make us stressed – another reason why the unhealthy foods and the alcohol are always at least two thirds of the way around the store.

Whereas many (most?) overweight people react to stress by eating comfort food, thin-thin people tend to be much more proactive, using meditation, mindfulness and holistic mind/body approaches like tai chi and yoga to actively manage stress. This allows them to deploy a response called "pause and plan" when faced with a stressful situation. In this way, thin-thin people are much better equipped to navigate supermarkets, restaurants and other tempting food outlets.

🏃 Habit eighteen: thin people don't eat emotionally

While overweight people will get into a comfort-eating pattern when they are stressed, or when their willpower weakens, thin-thin people simply do not eat for emotional reasons. Of course, thin-thin people are not saints who never put a foot wrong. The difference is in the way they react if they do.

Whereas overweight people beat themselves up for their perceived failure, thin-thin people are much kinder. Rather than scolding themselves (and getting even more miserable), they just remember that we are all human, we all slip up from time to time. Indeed, many thin-thin people use the opportunity to learn from their mistakes. For example, if they buy unhealthy food when they do their shop, they will review their actions and their state of mind to understand how this happened. This will give them greater control next time.

⛷ Habit nineteen: thin people eat slowly and mindfully (and banish distractions)

We often assume that overweight people enjoy food more than thin people, and that this helps to explain why they are thin. In fact, the opposite – at least in the way we behave – is true. Overweight people often eat with their minds on something else. Just check how often you eat in front of a screen or use your phone during a meal.

Overweight people may get through a large *quantity* of food, but they seldom enjoy the *quality.* Indeed, many of the sugary foods they eat act to dampen the taste buds, making most foods taste bland.

Thin-thin people are the very opposite of this. They are concerned with the quality of their food. Their tendency not to eat sugary or salty foods means that their taste buds are alive to the full flavour of the foods they eat. And when thin-thin people sit down for a meal (which they are most likely to do at a dining table), they focus their attention on eating, having banished all other potential distractions.

⚡ Habit twenty: thin people don't eat what they don't like

A corollary to thin-thin people's concern with the quality of their food is that they are much less likely to eat foods that they don't like.

Whereas an overweight people are likely to carry on eating food they don't enjoy, thin-thin people are much more likely to leave it on the plate. For example, because their taste buds are more sensitive to taste, on the occasions when they do opt for a dessert, thin-thin people will often find the flavour overpoweringly sweet and sickly. But rather than eating it anyway, they will leave it in favour of an alternative (such as a few squares of real chocolate).

⚡ Habit twenty two: thin people have a healthy attitude to waste

Thin-thin people are also less concerned about waste.

Many overweight people were taught not to leave food on their plates when they were children. This is particularly true of the baby-boomer generation whose parents went through the shortages of the 1930s and the Second World War. Culturally, they had learned that it was more important to eat more calories than to worry about putting on weight –

something that only affluent people were able to do until the 1960s.

As adults, many of us have internalised this desire not to waste food. The result is that we will often continue to eat food even if we feel full, simply to avoid wasting it.

Thin-thin people by contrast have learned that it is okay to leave food on your plate if you are full. Indeed, one common habit of thin-thin people is to throw their napkin onto any food still on their plate as a psychological device to prevent them picking at the leftovers.

𝓩 Habit twenty three: thin people don't apologise when they order

When we eat out, most of us simply order from the menu. The result is usually that we have to compromise by opting for the *healthiest* item that we can see when we should be choosing *healthy* options.

Thin-thin people will not do this, and they are unapologetic. When they order, they will ask for what they want irrespective of what the menu says. For example, they will ask for a burger without the bun, and salad without the dressing.

This is about learning to be assertive – if a restaurant wants your custom, they will provide the food you ask for. And if they won't, a thin-thin person will just get up and go elsewhere!

☰ Habit twenty four: thin people avoid high-sugar foods

It is difficult to know where to start when thinking about sugar. It is quite simply the single biggest cause of obesity around the world. No ifs, no buts, wherever you find obesity and the diseases collectively known as metabolic syndrome, you will find that a high sugar diet – and especially soda – was introduced around a decade previously[7].

Sugar is (albeit mildly) addictive – the more of it you have, the more of it you need. Perhaps most obviously this is experienced as a deadening of your sense of taste, leaving you needing ever sweeter foods. If you don't believe me, avoid sugar (and artificial sweeteners) for a week. See how this changes your sense of taste.

Unfortunately, the food industry adds sugar to almost all processed foods. And as there are more than 50 names for sugar, it is not easy to tell from the labels. However, thin-thin people actively avoid these foods. They not only avoid sugar, but also refined (white) carbohydrates, soda, and processed

---

[7] The seminal book on the danger of sugar is John Yudkin's (1972): *Pure, White And Deadly: How sugar is killing us and what we can do to stop it.*

foods. In this way, they minimise their exposure to sugar.

𝓩 Habit twenty five: thin people watch portion sizes

Most of us over-estimate the amount of food we need. This is particularly true for overweight people because the energy required just to carry the extra weight will leave you feeling hungry even after you have eaten a large meal. Nor is this helped by the food industry's tendency to offer large portions as standard. And in recent years the supermarkets have encouraged us to "buy one, get one free".

Thin-thin people are much more conservative in their portion sizes. At home they will use smaller plates so that a small portion looks bigger. Along with their other healthy habits, this helps them avoid over-eating.

𝓩 Habit twenty seven: thin people never eat before bedtime

The jury is out on whether the time of day you eat affects your weight. There is a theory that eating immediately before bed results in your body storing calories as fat instead of burning them (as you would when awake). However, there is little evidence for this.

It is more likely that people who eat immediately before bed experience disrupted sleep as their digestive system works through the night to process the unexpected meal. This, in turn, results in poor quality sleep and early waking, leaving them tired and more prone to overeat during the day (see habit 7).

Thin-thin people make a rule of not eating in the two to three hours before bed.

⚡ Habit twenty-eight: thin people treat themselves once a week

Where thin-thin people have a weakness for a particular unhealthy food, they use it to their advantage. Whether it is chocolate, cake, cheese, sweets or fries, they will use it as a reward (remember how important incentives and rewards are to willpower).

Whereas overweight people consume many of these "treat" foods as if they were part of a normal diet, thin-thin people will save them for special occasions or as a reward for achieving their goals during the week. Nor do these goals necessarily have to be food-related. For example, a reward for doing physical exercise might be a cup of coffee and a slice of cake at the end of the week[8].

---

[8] There is good evidence that deferring the reward helps to bolster and strengthen willpower in all areas of your life.

⚡ Habit twenty nine: thin people weigh themselves once a week

Psychologists have identified a human behaviour called "trading safety for peace of mind". What this means is we would prefer to ignore anything unpleasant rather than address it. At its extreme, this is why many victims of cancer fail to seek help at an early stage (when their cancer is curable) because they prefer the (temporary) peace of mind that comes from not knowing. It is also why the technicians at the Three Mile Island nuclear power station chose to believe there was a problem with their instruments rather than accept that the power station was going into meltdown.

Less extreme, but still dangerous at the personal level, many overweight people refuse to weigh themselves because they don't want to experience the anxiety and misery of finding that they have put on weight. Overweight people will often blame stores for selling them clothes that are "small for their size", or blame their washing powder for shrinking their clothes rather than acknowledge that they are putting on weight.

Thin-thin people understand that the temporary peace of mind that comes from not knowing your weight will soon be outweighed by the consequences of putting more weight on. So they make a habit of checking their weight around once every week[9].

🏃 Habit thirty: thin people intervene early

Overweight people fall into the trap of thinking that they will have much more willpower in future than they have in the present. This is a real problem because the future never arrives. We always live in the present. And if anything, constantly giving in to temptation today actually weakens willpower in the future.

So where overweight people are inclined to put off taking action, thin-thin people act immediately. They adjust their diet and engage in additional physical activity. After all, common sense tells you that it is much easier to lose a pound of weight now than it is to lose several pounds later on.

🏃 Habit thirty one: thin people keep their plans to themselves

A common and seriously annoying trait of overweight people when they are trying to lose

---

[9] Weight fluctuates during the day and from day to day. So there is a risk of becoming obsessive about fluctuations in your weight. It is much more important to measure the trend in your weight from week to week than to measure more often and end up worrying about fluctuations.

weight is they spend hours telling other people about the food they are/are not eating. This is often a way of substituting the *idea* of losing weight for the *practice*.

Thin-thin people do not talk about their weight loss practices. This isn't just because they *do* while others only *talk about* doing. It is also because telling others that you are trying to lose or manage your weight serves to put pressure on you to succeed. This pressure causes stress, and we have seen (habit 17) what stress does to your willpower.

🏃 Habit thirty two: thin people put themselves first

Many overweight people struggle because much of their lives involve meeting the needs of others. Whether looking after children, running a home or meeting the requirements of a stressful job, there just doesn't seem to be time left over to look after themselves.

Thin-thin people are much less compromising. This is particularly true when it comes to the food they eat, the physical activity they do, and the steps they take to manage stress.

⚡ Habit thirty three: thin people never food shop when they're hungry

Hunger is the single biggest trick in the supermarkets' psychological armoury. They know that the hungrier we are when we shop, the more likely we are to fill our trolleys with calorie-dense high-sugar and high-fat foods. This is so much so that many supermarkets will offer free sample food just to whet your appetite.

Thin-thin people understand that shopping on an empty stomach is dangerous. To combat this, they do two things:

- ○ Do one large shop each week (to cut the exposure to temptation[10]), and
- ○ Always shop after a meal.

This allows them to stick to buying those healthy foods on their list.

⚡ Habit thirty four: thin people limit their options

Thin-thin people deploy one of the most effective tricks of all when navigating supermarkets and restaurants – they limit their choice.

---

[10] Internet shopping *may* help curb temptation, but only if the items on your shopping list are healthy and you are not tempted by any of the supermarket's offers.

Whereas most overweight people shop chaotically – filling their trolleys with whatever items take their fancy – thin-thin people have a limited weekly menu of meals that they prepare from a relatively small list of healthy ingredients. Having got into this habit, they do not end up buying unhealthy food, even when they are sorely tempted.

The same goes for eating out. Where overweight people treat eating out as an adventure – in which they don't know what they are going to eat until they see the menu – thin-thin people plump for certainty; choosing the same restaurant(s) and the same healthy meal(s) every time.

🏃 Habit thirty five: thin people keep healthy food to hand (and banish unhealthy food)

Finally – and most important of all – thin-thin people create a food environment that they can control. They do this by making it very easy to access healthy foods while making it as difficult as possible to access unhealthy food.

For example, not having foods like chocolate, cake or crisps in the house means that if they want them, they are going to have to get in the car and drive to the shops to buy them. This allows them to exercise that all-important "pause and plan" response.

To complement this, they will also make it very easy to access something healthy like an apple or a banana, such as having these right next to their chair or workstation.

So their choice will be having an easy healthy snack or an unhealthy snack that involves a lot of hassle.

🏂 **Conclusion** 🏂

I hope I have shown that there is nothing accidental about weight gain and weight loss. By examining the habits of thin-thin people, and by contrasting these with the habits of overweight people, it is easy to understand why so many people struggle to lose weight, and all too often end up adding to their weight when they try.

Getting thin and *staying* thin is not about dieting. By their very nature, diets are temporary practices involving short-term goals. If you are serious about losing weight, you need to be in for the long haul.

The goals you set should be lifetime goals, like having more energy, avoiding illness as you get older, and living long enough to watch your grandchildren growing up. If you are serious about these goals, then you will realise that weight loss is about a profound change in your lifestyle. You need to think and act like a thin-thin person if you are going to succeed. That means making the 35 habits set out in this guide an integral part of your life.

Take small steps. The aim here is to move to a healthier lifestyle, not to set yourself up to fail. Choose those habits that appeal to you most to begin with. And please don't beat yourself up when you slip up. Remember, we are all only human, but we can learn from our mistakes.

Initially, you will need to practice the habits of being thin consciously. But eventually, if you stick with them they will become second nature. And the best time to start is right now.

So what are you waiting for?

🏄 About Life Surfing 🏄

Life Surfing is a Community Interest Company (a not-for-profit organisation: like a charity, but with paid managers) that was established to provide a coaching, mentoring and training approach for people experiencing common life problems that can cause stress, anxiety and depression.

Our mission is to help people learn to cope with life without the need to call on over-stretched health services that are better deployed to help people with severe and enduring mental illness.

Over the years we have found that there is a huge amount that people can do to develop their personal resources and to foster their own wellbeing. In most cases, the real need is for encouragement, support, knowledge and skills. This is what Life Surfing offers.

We have developed a range of training workshops, publications and a group programme to give you the knowledge and skills needed to address life's problems in a healthy way, and to promote long-term wellbeing.

We also provide 1-to-1 wellbeing coaching to help you take control of your personal wellbeing. These sessions are available in person or at a distance via Google+ or Skype.

For further information, please visit the Life Surfing website:

www.life-surfing.com

Or you can contact us:

0300 321 4514

info@life-surfing.com

⚡Other publications from Life Surfing ⚡

Life Surfing has published a growing range of wellbeing and self-help guides for anyone who is struggling with life's ups and downs, and anyone who wants to do more to help. Our publications are available from Amazon in paperback and Kindle formats - see the Life Surfing website for details.

- o *No More Panic: A Guide to overcoming panic attacks and recovering from panic disorder* This easy to digest, empowering and informative booklet explains how anyone can learn to manage and overcome panic attacks and panic disorder.

- o *Beating Anxiety: A Guide to Managing and Overcoming Anxiety Disorders.* This Life Surfing guide explains what anxiety is, how it is treated, and - crucially - what steps you can take to help yourself recover and sustain your personal wellbeing.

- o *Depression: A guide to managing and overcoming depression.* This Life Surfing Guide to depression provides you with an introduction to what depression is, how it is treated, and - crucially - what you can do to help yourself overcome the condition and create long-term personal wellbeing.

○ *Depression Workbook: 70 Self-help techniques for recovering from depression.* This book provides you with 70 self-help techniques covering the seven key areas of your personal wellbeing.

○ *Distress to De-stress: Understanding and managing stress in everyday life.* This Life Surfing guide explains what stress is, and - crucially - what healthy steps you can take to manage stress and promote long-term personal wellbeing. The guide includes 30 stress management techniques.

○ *Food for Mood: A guide to healthy eating for mental health.* In this Life Surfing guide we explain how mental health problems can impact on diet and how you can improve your diet by using foods from the helpful lists of good mood foods set out in the guide. We also provide some good mood food starter recipes for anyone who is relatively new to cooking.

○ *Getting to sleep: A guide to overcoming stress-related sleep problems.* With 1 in 3 of us experiencing stress-related insomnia, this important Life Surfing guide will give you a good understanding of sleep and - crucially - the steps you can take to improve the quality and duration of your sleep... night after night.

o *How to Help: A guide to helping someone manage mental distress.* In this Life Surfing guide, we explain what mental health and mental illness are, and - crucially - the steps that you can take to help someone experiencing mental health problems or mental illness.

o *Helping Hands: How to Help Someone Else Cope with Mental Health Problems.* Worried about the wellbeing of a relative, friend, colleague or client? Not sure what to do or worried you might say or do the wrong thing? *Helping Hands* will provide you with an understanding of wellbeing, and knowledge of mental illness, and will show you how you can help and support someone who has, or is at risk of developing, a mental health problem. *Helping Hands* also sets out a great deal of what has been learned about self-help and self-management strategies for recovery from mental illness over the last 25 years.